OSTEOPOROSIS DIET COOKBOOK

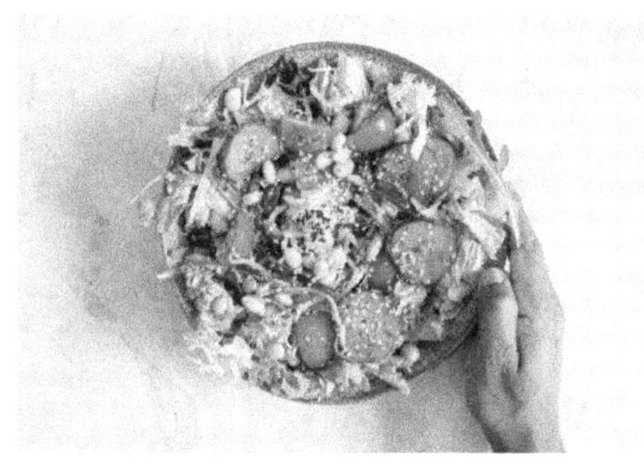

DR. JESSICA SMITH

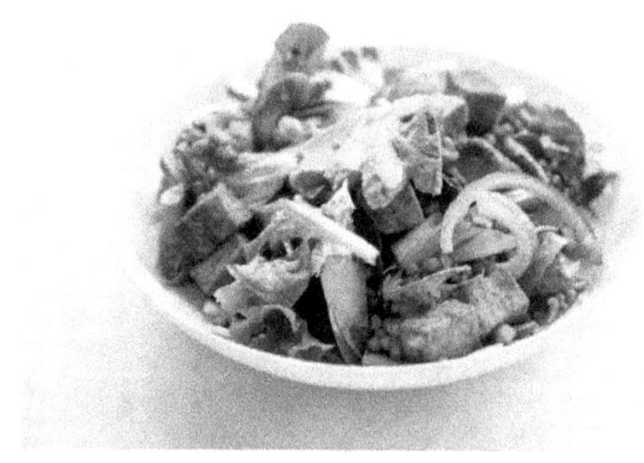

TABLE OF CONTENTS

CHAPTER ONE

How to Use this Cookbook

Understand the Basics: Begin by familiarizing yourself with the basics of an osteoporosis-friendly diet. This typically involves increasing calcium intake, consuming adequate vitamin D, getting enough protein, and reducing sodium intake.

Read the Introduction and Guidelines: Before diving into the recipes, read the introduction and guidelines sections of the cookbook.

This will provide valuable information on the principles of the osteoporosis diet, recommended daily allowances, and tips for meal planning.

Take Stock of Ingredients: Review the ingredient lists of various recipes in the cookbook. Make a list of ingredients you need to stock up on, paying particular attention to calcium-rich foods like dairy products, leafy greens, and fortified foods.

Plan Your Meals: Plan your meals for the week ahead based on the recipes in the cookbook.

Aim for a balanced diet that includes a variety of foods rich in calcium, vitamin D, magnesium, and other bone-healthy nutrients.

Experiment with Recipes: Don't be afraid to experiment with different recipes from the cookbook. Try incorporating new flavors and ingredients into your meals to keep things interesting and enjoyable.

Follow Cooking Instructions Carefully: When preparing recipes from the cookbook, be sure to follow the cooking instructions carefully. Pay attention to portion sizes and cooking methods to ensure that you're getting the most nutritional benefit from each meal.

Be Mindful of Nutrient Content: Pay attention to the nutrient content of each recipe, particularly calcium, vitamin D, and protein. Make adjustments to your meal plan as needed to ensure that you're meeting your daily nutritional requirements.

Stay Hydrated: Don't forget the importance of staying hydrated for bone health. Drink plenty of water throughout the day, and consider incorporating bone-healthy beverages like milk, fortified orange juice, or herbal teas into your routine.

Monitor Your Progress: Keep track of how you feel as you follow the osteoporosis diet using the cookbook. Monitor any changes in your bone health, energy levels, and overall well-being. If you have any concerns or questions, don't hesitate to consult with a healthcare professional.

Understanding Osteoporosis Diet

Understanding the osteoporosis diet involves grasping the fundamental principles of nutrition that support bone health.

Osteoporosis, a condition characterized by weakened bones, necessitates a dietary approach rich in specific nutrients vital for bone strength and density. Calcium stands as a cornerstone, essential for bone mineralization and maintenance.

Foods such as dairy products, leafy greens, tofu, and fortified foods serve as excellent calcium sources. Equally crucial is vitamin D, which aids in calcium absorption.

Fatty fish, fortified dairy, egg yolks, and sunlight exposure contribute to vitamin D intake.

Protein plays a vital role in bone health, assisting in bone formation and repair. Lean meats, poultry, fish, beans, and nuts are excellent protein sources. Conversely, excessive sodium intake should be minimized, as it can lead to calcium loss from bones.

Understanding portion sizes and balanced meals is key to crafting an osteoporosis-friendly diet. It involves incorporating a variety of nutrient-dense foods while moderating intake of foods high in saturated fats and sugars, which may negatively impact bone health.

Hydration is essential, as adequate water intake supports overall health and may help prevent bone mineral loss.

Comprehending the osteoporosis diet involves recognizing the significance of a well-rounded, nutrient-rich eating pattern to promote optimal bone health and reduce the risk of fractures.

Benefits of Osteoporosis Diet

The benefits of an osteoporosis diet extend far beyond mere bone health, impacting overall well-being and quality of life. By adhering to a diet rich in nutrients crucial for bone strength, individuals can experience several advantages:

Improved Bone Health: A diet focused on osteoporosis prevention and management provides essential nutrients like calcium, vitamin D, magnesium, and protein, promoting bone mineralization, density, and strength. This reduces the risk of fractures and slows down bone loss associated with osteoporosis.

Enhanced Muscle Health: A balanced diet rich in protein supports muscle health and function. Strong muscles can provide better support to bones, reducing the risk of falls and fractures.

Optimized Nutrient Intake: Following an osteoporosis diet ensures adequate intake of key nutrients necessary for bone health, such as calcium and vitamin D, as well as other vital nutrients like potassium, magnesium, and vitamin K.

Reduced Risk of Chronic Diseases: Many foods beneficial for bone health, such as fruits, vegetables, and whole grains, are also associated with a lower risk of chronic diseases like heart disease, diabetes, and certain cancers.

Improved Overall Health: A diet focused on osteoporosis prevention typically emphasizes whole, nutrient-dense foods while minimizing processed foods high in unhealthy fats and sugars. This can lead to improved overall health, including better weight management, blood sugar control, and cholesterol levels.

Enhanced Quality of Life: By reducing the risk of fractures and maintaining overall health, an osteoporosis diet can contribute to a higher quality of life, allowing individuals to remain active, independent, and engaged in daily activities for longer.

Guidelines for Osteoporosis Diet

When navigating an osteoporosis diet, it's essential to adhere to specific guidelines aimed at promoting bone health and reducing the risk of fractures.

Here are some key guidelines to consider:

Calcium-Rich Foods: Incorporate foods rich in calcium into your daily diet. Dairy products like milk, yogurt, and cheese are traditional sources, but non-dairy options such as fortified plant-based milks, tofu, almonds, and leafy greens like kale and spinach are also excellent choices.

Adequate Vitamin D Intake: Ensure sufficient vitamin D intake to support calcium absorption and bone health.

Exposure to sunlight, fortified foods like cereal and orange juice, fatty fish like salmon and mackerel, and supplements if necessary can help meet your vitamin D needs.

Balanced Diet: Aim for a balanced diet that includes a variety of nutrient-dense foods, such as fruits, vegetables, whole grains, lean proteins, and healthy fats. This provides essential vitamins and minerals necessary for overall health and bone strength.

Limit Sodium and Caffeine: Reduce consumption of foods high in sodium and caffeine, as they can contribute to calcium loss from bones. Be mindful of processed foods, salty snacks, and caffeinated beverages like coffee and soda.

Moderate Alcohol Consumption: Limit alcohol intake, as excessive alcohol consumption can weaken bones and increase the risk of fractures. Stick to moderate amounts, if any, and consider healthier alternatives like water or herbal tea.

Regular Physical Activity: Engage in weight-bearing exercises like walking, jogging, dancing, or strength training regularly to build and maintain bone density. Incorporate balance and flexibility exercises to reduce the risk of falls.

Quit Smoking: If you smoke, quitting can benefit bone health. Smoking is linked to decreased bone density and an increased risk of fractures, so seek support and resources to quit smoking if needed.

Regular Bone Density Tests: Consider regular bone density tests as recommended by your healthcare provider to monitor your bone health and make necessary adjustments to your diet and lifestyle.

You can effectively support your bone health and reduce the risk of osteoporosis-related complications.

Always consult with a healthcare professional or registered dietitian for personalized advice tailored to your specific needs and health status.

CHAPTER TWO

1: Spinach and Feta Omelette

Ingredients:

- 2 eggs
- 1 cup fresh spinach, chopped
- 2 tablespoons crumbled feta cheese
- Salt and pepper to taste
- 1 teaspoon olive oil

Instructions:

- In a small bowl, whisk together the eggs until well beaten. Season with salt and pepper.
- Heat olive oil in a non-stick skillet over medium heat.
- Add chopped spinach to the skillet and sauté for 1-2 minutes until wilted.
- Pour the beaten eggs over the spinach in the skillet. Allow the eggs to cook for 1-2 minutes until the edges start to set.

- Sprinkle crumbled feta cheese over one half of the omelette.
- Using a spatula, carefully fold the other half of the omelette over the cheese.
- Cook for another 1-2 minutes until the cheese is melted and the eggs are fully cooked.
- Slide the omelette onto a plate and serve hot.

Health Benefits:

- This omelette is packed with calcium from the spinach and feta cheese, providing essential nutrients for bone health.
- The eggs also contribute protein, while spinach adds fiber and vitamins.

Preparation Time: Approximately 10 minutes.

2: Greek Yogurt Parfait

Ingredients:

- 1 cup plain Greek yogurt
- 1/2 cup mixed berries (such as strawberries, blueberries, raspberries)
- 2 tablespoons chopped walnuts

- 1 tablespoon honey or maple syrup (optional)

Instructions:

- In a glass or bowl, layer half of the Greek yogurt.
- Add half of the mixed berries on top of the yogurt.
- Sprinkle half of the chopped walnuts over the berries.
- Repeat the layers with the remaining yogurt, berries, and walnuts.
- Drizzle honey or maple syrup over the top if desired.
- Serve immediately or refrigerate until ready to eat.

Health Benefits:

- This Greek yogurt parfait is rich in calcium and protein from the yogurt, as well as antioxidants and vitamins from the mixed berries.
- Walnuts provide omega-3 fatty acids, which are beneficial for bone health.

Preparation Time: Approximately 5 minutes.

3: Overnight Oats with Almond Butter and Banana

Ingredients:

- 1/2 cup rolled oats
- 1/2 cup almond milk (or any milk of your choice)
- 1 tablespoon almond butter
- 1/2 ripe banana, mashed
- 1 tablespoon chia seeds (optional)
- 1 teaspoon honey or maple syrup (optional)
- Sliced banana and chopped almonds for topping

Instructions:

- In a mason jar or a bowl, combine rolled oats, almond milk, mashed banana, almond butter, chia seeds (if using), and honey or maple syrup (if desired). Stir well to combine.
- Cover the jar or bowl and refrigerate overnight, or for at least 4 hours, to allow the oats to soak and soften.
- When ready to serve, give the oats a stir and add a splash of milk if desired to reach your desired consistency.

- Top with sliced banana and chopped almonds before serving.

Health Benefits:

- This breakfast is rich in calcium from the almond milk, almond butter, and chia seeds.
- Oats provide fiber, while bananas offer potassium and other essential vitamins and minerals.

Preparation Time: Approximately 5 minutes (plus chilling time).

4: Avocado Toast with Smoked Salmon

Ingredients:

- 2 slices whole grain bread
- 1 ripe avocado
- Juice of 1/2 lemon
- Salt and pepper to taste
- 2 ounces smoked salmon
- Optional toppings: sliced tomato, microgreens, red onion

Instructions:

- Toast the slices of whole grain bread until golden brown.
- In a small bowl, mash the ripe avocado with lemon juice, salt, and pepper until smooth.
- Spread the mashed avocado evenly onto the toasted bread slices.
- Top each slice with smoked salmon.
- Add optional toppings such as sliced tomato, microgreens, or red onion if desired.
- Serve immediately.

Health Benefits:

- This avocado toast is packed with nutrients beneficial for bone health, including calcium from the whole grain bread and healthy fats from avocado and salmon.
- Avocado also provides potassium and vitamin K.

Preparation Time: Approximately 10 minutes.

Ingredients:

- 1/2 cup cooked quinoa
- 1/2 cup plain Greek yogurt
- 1/4 cup mixed berries (such as strawberries, blueberries, raspberries)
- 1 tablespoon honey or maple syrup
- 1 tablespoon chopped almonds or walnuts
- 1/2 teaspoon ground cinnamon (optional)

Instructions:

- In a bowl, layer cooked quinoa as the base.
- Top the quinoa with plain Greek yogurt.
- Add mixed berries on top of the yogurt.
- Drizzle honey or maple syrup over the berries.
- Sprinkle chopped almonds or walnuts on top.
- Optionally, sprinkle ground cinnamon over the entire bowl for added flavor.
- Serve immediately.

Health Benefits:

- This breakfast bowl is rich in calcium and protein from the Greek yogurt, as well as fiber and other essential nutrients from quinoa and berries.
- Nuts provide healthy fats and additional protein.

Preparation Time: Approximately 15 minutes (if quinoa is already cooked).

6: Green Smoothie

Ingredients:

- 1 cup fresh spinach leaves
- 1/2 ripe banana
- 1/2 cup plain Greek yogurt
- 1/2 cup almond milk (or any milk of your choice)
- 1 tablespoon almond butter or peanut butter
- 1 tablespoon chia seeds
- Optional: honey or maple syrup to taste
- Ice cubes (optional)

Instructions:

- In a blender, combine fresh spinach leaves, banana, Greek yogurt, almond milk, almond butter, and chia seeds.
- Optionally, add honey or maple syrup for sweetness, if desired.
- Blend until smooth and creamy.
- Add ice cubes if you prefer a colder smoothie and blend again until well combined.
- Pour the smoothie into a glass and serve immediately.

Health Benefits:

- This green smoothie is packed with calcium from spinach and Greek yogurt, as well as potassium and other vitamins and minerals from banana.
- Chia seeds add omega-3 fatty acids and fiber.

Preparation Time: Approximately 5 minutes.

7: Chia Seed Pudding

Ingredients:

- 1/4 cup chia seeds
- 1 cup almond milk (or any milk of your choice)

- 1/2 teaspoon vanilla extract

- 1 tablespoon honey or maple syrup

- Fresh fruit for topping (such as berries, sliced banana)

- Optional: chopped nuts or shredded coconut for topping

Instructions:

- In a bowl or jar, mix together chia seeds, almond milk, vanilla extract, and honey or maple syrup.

- Stir well to combine, ensuring that the chia seeds are evenly distributed.

- Cover the bowl or jar and refrigerate for at least 2 hours, or overnight, until the mixture thickens into a pudding-like consistency.

- Once the chia seed pudding is set, give it a stir and divide it into serving bowls.

- Top each serving with fresh fruit and optional toppings such as chopped nuts or shredded coconut.

- Serve chilled and enjoy!

Health Benefits:

- Chia seeds are rich in calcium, fiber, and omega-3 fatty acids, making them an excellent addition to the osteoporosis diet. Almond milk provides additional calcium, while fresh fruit adds vitamins and antioxidants.

Preparation Time: Approximately 5 minutes (plus chilling time).

8: Veggie and Cheese Breakfast Quesadilla

Ingredients:

- 2 small whole wheat tortillas
- 1/2 cup shredded cheese (such as cheddar or mozzarella)
- 1/4 cup diced bell peppers (any color)
- 1/4 cup diced tomatoes
- 2 tablespoons diced red onion
- 1/4 cup chopped spinach
- Optional: salsa or avocado for serving

Instructions:

- Heat a non-stick skillet over medium heat.

- Place one tortilla in the skillet and sprinkle half of the shredded cheese evenly over the tortilla.
- Layer diced bell peppers, tomatoes, red onion, and chopped spinach on top of the cheese.
- Sprinkle the remaining cheese over the vegetables.
- Place the second tortilla on top to cover the filling, pressing down gently.
- Cook the quesadilla for 2-3 minutes on each side, or until the tortillas are golden brown and the cheese is melted.
- Remove the quesadilla from the skillet and let it cool for a minute before slicing into wedges.
- Serve with salsa or avocado if desired.

Health Benefits:

- This breakfast quesadilla is a great way to incorporate vegetables into your morning meal.
- Bell peppers, tomatoes, onions, and spinach provide vitamins, minerals, and antioxidants, while whole wheat tortillas add fiber.

Preparation Time: Approximately 10 minutes.

9: Almond Butter and Banana Smoothie Bowl

Ingredients:

- 1 ripe banana
- 1/4 cup almond butter
- 1/2 cup almond milk (or any milk of your choice)
- 1/2 cup plain Greek yogurt
- 1 tablespoon honey or maple syrup
- 1/2 cup rolled oats
- Toppings: sliced banana, chopped almonds, chia seeds, shredded coconut

Instructions:

- In a blender, combine the ripe banana, almond butter, almond milk, Greek yogurt, honey or maple syrup, and rolled oats.
- Blend until smooth and creamy, adding more almond milk if needed to reach your desired consistency.
- Pour the smoothie into a bowl.
- Top with sliced banana, chopped almonds, chia seeds, and shredded coconut.
- Serve immediately and enjoy with a spoon!

Health Benefits:

- This smoothie bowl is rich in calcium, protein, and healthy fats from almond butter and Greek yogurt.
- Bananas provide potassium and fiber, while oats add additional fiber and nutrients.

Preparation Time: Approximately 5 minutes.

10: Sweet Potato Breakfast Hash

Ingredients:

- 1 medium sweet potato, peeled and diced
- 1/2 red bell pepper, diced
- 1/2 green bell pepper, diced
- 1/4 red onion, diced
- 2 tablespoons olive oil
- 1 teaspoon paprika
- 1/2 teaspoon garlic powder
- Salt and pepper to taste
- 2 eggs
- Optional: chopped fresh parsley or cilantro for garnish

Instructions:

- Heat olive oil in a skillet over medium heat.
- Add diced sweet potato to the skillet and cook for 5-7 minutes, stirring occasionally, until slightly softened.
- Add diced bell peppers and red onion to the skillet. Cook for another 5-7 minutes, until vegetables are tender and lightly browned.
- Season the vegetables with paprika, garlic powder, salt, and pepper. Stir to combine.
- Create two wells in the hash mixture and crack an egg into each well.
- Cover the skillet and cook for 3-5 minutes, or until the eggs are cooked to your desired doneness.
- Remove the skillet from heat and garnish with chopped fresh parsley or cilantro if desired.
- Divide the breakfast hash onto plates and serve hot.

Health Benefits:

- Sweet potatoes are rich in vitamin C, potassium, and fiber, while bell peppers and onions provide additional vitamins and antioxidants.

- Eggs contribute protein and essential nutrients.

Preparation Time: Approximately 20 minutes.

1: Salmon and Quinoa Salad

Ingredients:

- 1 cup cooked quinoa
- 4 ounces cooked salmon, flaked
- 1 cup mixed salad greens
- 1/2 cup cherry tomatoes, halved
- 1/4 cup cucumber, diced
- 1/4 cup red bell pepper, diced
- 2 tablespoons sliced almonds
- 1 tablespoon olive oil
- 1 tablespoon lemon juice
- Salt and pepper to taste

Instructions:

- In a large bowl, combine the cooked quinoa, flaked salmon, mixed salad greens, cherry tomatoes, cucumber, red bell pepper, and sliced almonds.

- Drizzle olive oil and lemon juice over the salad.

- Season with salt and pepper to taste.

- Toss the salad gently until all ingredients are evenly coated with the dressing.

- Divide the salad into serving bowls.

- Serve immediately and enjoy!

Health Benefits:

- This salad is rich in calcium, protein, and omega-3 fatty acids from salmon, which are essential for bone health.

- Quinoa provides additional protein and fiber, while vegetables add vitamins, minerals, and antioxidants.

Preparation Time: Approximately 20 minutes (if quinoa and salmon are already cooked).

2: Turkey and Avocado Wrap

Ingredients:

- 1 whole grain tortilla or wrap

- 2 slices cooked turkey breast

- 1/4 avocado, sliced

- 1/4 cup shredded lettuce

- 2 slices tomato

- 1 tablespoon hummus or Greek yogurt spread

- Optional: sliced cucumber, shredded carrot, sprouts

Instructions:

- Lay the whole grain tortilla or wrap on a flat surface.

- Spread hummus or Greek yogurt spread evenly over the tortilla.

- Layer cooked turkey breast, sliced avocado, shredded lettuce, tomato slices, and any additional toppings (such as sliced cucumber, shredded carrot, or sprouts) on top of the spread.

- Roll up the tortilla tightly into a wrap, tucking in the sides as you go.

- Slice the wrap in half diagonally.

- Serve immediately, or wrap in foil or parchment paper for later.

Health Benefits:

- This turkey and avocado wrap is a balanced meal providing protein, healthy fats, and fiber.

- Turkey is a lean source of protein, while avocado offers heart-healthy monounsaturated fats.
- Whole grain tortillas provide fiber, contributing to overall digestive health.

Preparation Time: Approximately 10 minutes.

3: Lentil and Vegetable Soup

Ingredients:

- 1 cup dried green lentils, rinsed and drained
- 4 cups vegetable broth
- 1 onion, chopped
- 2 carrots, diced
- 2 celery stalks, diced
- 2 cloves garlic, minced
- 1 teaspoon dried thyme
- 1 teaspoon dried oregano
- Salt and pepper to taste
- 2 cups chopped spinach or kale
- Juice of 1 lemon
- Optional: chopped fresh parsley for garnish

Instructions:

- In a large pot, combine the dried lentils, vegetable broth, chopped onion, diced carrots, diced celery, minced garlic, dried thyme, dried oregano, salt, and pepper.
- Bring the mixture to a boil over medium-high heat.
- Reduce the heat to low, cover, and simmer for 20-25 minutes, or until the lentils and vegetables are tender.
- Stir in the chopped spinach or kale and lemon juice.
- Cook for an additional 5 minutes until the greens are wilted.
- Taste and adjust seasoning if needed.
- Ladle the soup into bowls and garnish with chopped fresh parsley if desired.
- Serve hot and enjoy!

Health Benefits:

- This lentil and vegetable soup is rich in plant-based protein, fiber, vitamins, and minerals.
- Lentils are high in folate, iron, and potassium, while vegetables provide essential nutrients for bone health.

Preparation Time: Approximately 40 minutes.

4: Chicken and Quinoa Stuffed Bell Peppers

Ingredients:

- 4 bell peppers, any color
- 1 cup cooked quinoa
- 1 cup cooked chicken breast, shredded
- 1/2 cup black beans, rinsed and drained
- 1/2 cup corn kernels
- 1/2 cup diced tomatoes
- 1/4 cup diced red onion
- 1 teaspoon chili powder
- 1/2 teaspoon cumin
- Salt and pepper to taste
- 1/2 cup shredded cheese (such as cheddar or mozzarella)
- Optional: chopped fresh cilantro for garnish

Instructions:

- Preheat the oven to 375°F (190°C). Grease a baking dish with olive oil.

- Cut the tops off the bell peppers and remove the seeds and membranes.
- In a large bowl, combine the cooked quinoa, shredded chicken breast, black beans, corn kernels, diced tomatoes, diced red onion, chili powder, cumin, salt, and pepper.
- Spoon the quinoa and chicken mixture into each bell pepper until they are filled to the top.
- Place the stuffed bell peppers in the prepared baking dish.
- Sprinkle shredded cheese evenly over the top of each stuffed pepper.
- Cover the baking dish with foil and bake in the preheated oven for 25-30 minutes, or until the peppers are tender and the filling is heated through.
- Remove the foil and bake for an additional 5 minutes, or until the cheese is melted and bubbly.
- Remove from the oven and let cool for a few minutes before serving.
- Garnish with chopped fresh cilantro if desired.
- Serve hot and enjoy!

Health Benefits:

- These stuffed bell peppers are packed with protein from the chicken and quinoa, as well as fiber and nutrients from the vegetables.
- Bell peppers are also rich in vitamin C, which aids in collagen production and bone health.

Preparation Time: Approximately 45 minutes.

5: Tofu and Vegetable Stir-Fry

Ingredients:

- 1 block (14 oz) extra-firm tofu, pressed and cubed
- 2 tablespoons soy sauce (or tamari for gluten-free option)
- 1 tablespoon sesame oil
- 2 cloves garlic, minced
- 1 teaspoon grated ginger
- 2 cups mixed vegetables (such as bell peppers, broccoli, carrots, snap peas)
- Cooked brown rice or quinoa for serving
- Optional garnish: sliced green onions, sesame seeds

Instructions:

- In a bowl, combine cubed tofu with soy sauce, sesame oil, minced garlic, and grated ginger. Let marinate for 15-20 minutes.
- Heat a large skillet or wok over medium-high heat. Add marinated tofu and cook until golden brown on all sides, about 5-7 minutes. Remove tofu from the skillet and set aside.
- In the same skillet, add mixed vegetables and stir-fry until tender-crisp, about 5-7 minutes.
- Return cooked tofu to the skillet with the vegetables and toss to combine.
- Serve the tofu and vegetable stir-fry over cooked brown rice or quinoa.
- Garnish with sliced green onions and sesame seeds, if desired.
- Enjoy hot!

Health Benefits:

- This tofu and vegetable stir-fry is a great source of plant-based protein from tofu and fiber-rich vegetables.

- Tofu is also rich in calcium, while vegetables provide essential vitamins and minerals necessary for bone health.

Preparation Time: Approximately 30 minutes.

6: Spinach and Chickpea Salad

Ingredients:

- 2 cups fresh spinach leaves
- 1/2 cup cooked chickpeas (canned, rinsed, and drained)
- 1/4 cup diced cucumber
- 1/4 cup halved cherry tomatoes
- 1/4 cup sliced red onion
- 2 tablespoons crumbled feta cheese (optional)
- 1 tablespoon extra-virgin olive oil
- 1 tablespoon balsamic vinegar
- Salt and pepper to taste

Instructions:

- In a large bowl, combine fresh spinach leaves, cooked chickpeas, diced cucumber, halved cherry tomatoes, sliced red onion, and crumbled feta cheese (if using).

- Drizzle extra-virgin olive oil and balsamic vinegar over the salad.
- Season with salt and pepper to taste.
- Toss the salad gently until all ingredients are evenly coated with the dressing.
- Divide the salad into serving bowls.
- Enjoy as a light and refreshing lunch option!

Health Benefits:

- This spinach and chickpea salad is rich in calcium, protein, and fiber.
- Spinach is a great source of bone-healthy nutrients, while chickpeas provide plant-based protein and fiber.
- The salad is also packed with vitamins, minerals, and antioxidants from vegetables.

Preparation Time: Approximately 15 minutes.

7: Mediterranean Quinoa Salad

Ingredients:

- 1 cup cooked quinoa
- 1 cup diced cucumber
- 1 cup halved cherry tomatoes
- 1/2 cup diced red bell pepper
- 1/4 cup chopped Kalamata olives
- 1/4 cup crumbled feta cheese
- 2 tablespoons chopped fresh parsley
- 2 tablespoons extra-virgin olive oil
- 1 tablespoon lemon juice
- 1 teaspoon dried oregano
- Salt and pepper to taste

Instructions:

- In a large bowl, combine cooked quinoa, diced cucumber, halved cherry tomatoes, diced red bell pepper, chopped Kalamata olives, crumbled feta cheese, and chopped fresh parsley.

- In a small bowl, whisk together extra-virgin olive oil, lemon juice, dried oregano, salt, and pepper to make the dressing.

- Pour the dressing over the quinoa salad and toss gently to coat all ingredients.
- Taste and adjust seasoning if needed.
- Serve immediately, or refrigerate for later.
- Enjoy this refreshing Mediterranean-inspired salad!

Health Benefits:

- This quinoa salad is loaded with nutrients beneficial for bone health, including calcium from the feta cheese and quinoa, as well as vitamins and antioxidants from the vegetables.
- Olive oil provides healthy fats, while olives add flavor and additional nutrients.

Preparation Time: Approximately 20 minutes.

8: Grilled Chicken Caesar Wrap

Ingredients:

- 1 whole grain tortilla or wrap
- 4 ounces grilled chicken breast, sliced
- 1 cup chopped romaine lettuce
- 2 tablespoons grated Parmesan cheese

- 2 tablespoons Caesar dressing (homemade or store-bought)
- Optional: diced tomatoes, croutons

Instructions:

- Lay the whole grain tortilla or wrap on a flat surface.
- Arrange sliced grilled chicken breast in the center of the tortilla.
- Top with chopped romaine lettuce, grated Parmesan cheese, and Caesar dressing.
- Add optional diced tomatoes and croutons if desired.
- Roll up the tortilla tightly into a wrap, tucking in the sides as you go.
- Slice the wrap in half diagonally.
- Serve immediately, or wrap in foil or parchment paper for later.
- Enjoy this delicious and satisfying chicken Caesar wrap!

Health Benefits:

- This grilled chicken Caesar wrap offers a balanced combination of protein from chicken, fiber from whole grain tortilla and vegetables, and calcium from Parmesan cheese. Romaine lettuce is also rich in vitamin K, which supports bone health.

Preparation Time: Approximately 15 minutes.

9: Spinach and White Bean Salad

Ingredients:

- 2 cups fresh spinach leaves
- 1 cup cooked white beans (cannellini beans), rinsed and drained
- 1/2 cup diced cucumber
- 1/2 cup diced red bell pepper
- 1/4 cup sliced red onion
- 2 tablespoons chopped fresh basil
- 2 tablespoons extra-virgin olive oil
- 1 tablespoon balsamic vinegar
- Salt and pepper to taste
- Optional: crumbled goat cheese or feta cheese

Instructions:

- In a large bowl, combine fresh spinach leaves, cooked white beans, diced cucumber, diced red bell pepper, sliced red onion, and chopped fresh basil.
- In a small bowl, whisk together extra-virgin olive oil, balsamic vinegar, salt, and pepper to make the dressing.
- Pour the dressing over the salad and toss gently to coat all ingredients.
- Taste and adjust seasoning if needed.
- Sprinkle crumbled goat cheese or feta cheese over the salad, if desired.
- Serve immediately as a light and nutritious lunch option!

Health Benefits:

- This spinach and white bean salad is packed with fiber, protein, vitamins, and minerals.
- White beans provide plant-based protein and calcium, while spinach offers essential nutrients like vitamin K and magnesium for bone health.

- Olive oil provides heart-healthy fats, and vegetables contribute antioxidants.

Preparation Time: Approximately 15 minutes.

10: Vegetable and Lentil Soup

Ingredients:

- 1 cup dried green lentils, rinsed and drained
- 4 cups vegetable broth
- 1 onion, chopped
- 2 carrots, diced
- 2 celery stalks, diced
- 2 cloves garlic, minced
- 1 teaspoon dried thyme
- 1 teaspoon dried rosemary
- Salt and pepper to taste
- 2 cups chopped kale or spinach
- Juice of 1 lemon
- Optional: grated Parmesan cheese for garnish

Instructions:

- In a large pot, combine dried lentils, vegetable broth, chopped onion, diced carrots, diced celery, minced garlic, dried thyme, dried rosemary, salt, and pepper.
- Bring the mixture to a boil over medium-high heat.
- Reduce the heat to low, cover, and simmer for 20-25 minutes, or until the lentils and vegetables are tender.
- Stir in chopped kale or spinach and lemon juice.
- Cook for an additional 5 minutes until the greens are wilted.
- Taste and adjust seasoning if needed.
- Ladle the soup into bowls and garnish with grated Parmesan cheese, if desired.
- Serve hot and enjoy this comforting and nourishing soup!

Health Benefits:

- This vegetable and lentil soup is a nutrient-rich meal loaded with fiber, protein, vitamins, and minerals.
- Lentils provide plant-based protein and iron, while vegetables offer antioxidants and essential nutrients

for bone health. Kale or spinach adds calcium and vitamin K.

Preparation Time: Approximately 40 minutes.

Osteoporosis Diet Dinner Recipes

1: Baked Salmon with Asparagus

Ingredients:

- 2 salmon fillets (about 6 ounces each)
- 1 bunch asparagus, trimmed
- 2 tablespoons olive oil
- 2 cloves garlic, minced
- 1 teaspoon lemon zest
- 1 tablespoon lemon juice
- Salt and pepper to taste
- Optional: chopped fresh parsley for garnish

Instructions:

- Preheat the oven to 400°F (200°C). Line a baking sheet with parchment paper.
- Place the salmon fillets on one side of the prepared baking sheet and arrange the trimmed asparagus on the other side.

- In a small bowl, whisk together olive oil, minced garlic, lemon zest, lemon juice, salt, and pepper.

- Drizzle the olive oil mixture over the salmon and asparagus, tossing the asparagus to coat evenly.

- Bake in the preheated oven for 12-15 minutes, or until the salmon is cooked through and flakes easily with a fork, and the asparagus is tender-crisp.

- Remove from the oven and garnish with chopped fresh parsley, if desired.

- Serve hot and enjoy this flavorful and nutritious dinner!

Health Benefits:

- This baked salmon with asparagus is rich in omega-3 fatty acids, protein, and calcium.

- Salmon is an excellent source of vitamin D and omega-3s, both of which are essential for bone health.

- Asparagus provides additional vitamins and minerals, including vitamin K and folate.

Preparation Time: Approximately 20 minutes.

2: Quinoa Stuffed Bell Peppers

Ingredients:

- 4 large bell peppers, any color
- 1 cup cooked quinoa
- 1 cup cooked black beans, rinsed and drained
- 1 cup diced tomatoes
- 1/2 cup corn kernels
- 1/4 cup diced red onion
- 1 teaspoon chili powder
- 1/2 teaspoon ground cumin
- Salt and pepper to taste
- 1/2 cup shredded cheese (such as cheddar or mozzarella)
- Optional: chopped fresh cilantro for garnish

Instructions:

- Preheat the oven to 375°F (190°C). Grease a baking dish with olive oil.
- Cut the tops off the bell peppers and remove the seeds and membranes.

- In a large bowl, combine cooked quinoa, black beans, diced tomatoes, corn kernels, diced red onion, chili powder, ground cumin, salt, and pepper.
- Spoon the quinoa mixture evenly into each bell pepper until they are filled to the top.
- Place the stuffed bell peppers in the prepared baking dish.
- Sprinkle shredded cheese evenly over the top of each stuffed pepper.
- Cover the baking dish with foil and bake in the preheated oven for 25-30 minutes, or until the peppers are tender and the filling is heated through.
- Remove the foil and bake for an additional 5 minutes, or until the cheese is melted and bubbly.
- Remove from the oven and let cool for a few minutes before serving.
- Garnish with chopped fresh cilantro if desired.
- Serve hot and enjoy this wholesome and satisfying dinner!

Health Benefits:

- These quinoa stuffed bell peppers are packed with protein, fiber, vitamins, and minerals.
- Quinoa and black beans provide plant-based protein and calcium, while bell peppers offer vitamin C and antioxidants.
- The dish is also low in calories and high in nutrients, making it an excellent choice for bone health.

Preparation Time: Approximately 45 minutes.

3: Veggie and Tofu Stir-Fry

Ingredients:

- 1 block (14 oz) extra-firm tofu, pressed and cubed
- 2 tablespoons soy sauce (or tamari for gluten-free option)
- 2 tablespoons hoisin sauce
- 1 tablespoon rice vinegar
- 1 tablespoon sesame oil
- 2 cloves garlic, minced
- 1 teaspoon grated ginger

- 2 cups mixed vegetables (such as bell peppers, broccoli, carrots, snap peas)
- Cooked brown rice or quinoa for serving
- Optional garnish: sliced green onions, sesame seeds

Instructions:

- In a bowl, combine cubed tofu with soy sauce and let marinate for 15-20 minutes.
- In a small bowl, mix hoisin sauce, rice vinegar, and sesame oil to make the sauce.
- Heat a large skillet or wok over medium-high heat. Add marinated tofu and cook until golden brown on all sides, about 5-7 minutes. Remove tofu from the skillet and set aside.
- In the same skillet, add minced garlic and grated ginger. Stir-fry for 1 minute until fragrant.
- Add mixed vegetables to the skillet and stir-fry until tender-crisp, about 5-7 minutes.
- Return cooked tofu to the skillet and pour the sauce over the tofu and vegetables. Toss to combine and heat through.

- Serve the veggie and tofu stir-fry over cooked brown rice or quinoa.

- Garnish with sliced green onions and sesame seeds, if desired.

- Enjoy this flavorful and nutritious stir-fry!

Health Benefits:

- This veggie and tofu stir-fry is rich in plant-based protein, fiber, vitamins, and minerals.

- Tofu provides calcium and protein, while mixed vegetables offer a variety of nutrients essential for bone health.

- Brown rice or quinoa adds complex carbohydrates and additional fiber.

Preparation Time: Approximately 30 minutes.

4: Chicken and Vegetable Skewers

Ingredients:

- 2 boneless, skinless chicken breasts, cut into cubes
- 2 bell peppers (any color), cut into chunks
- 1 zucchini, sliced into rounds
- 1 yellow squash, sliced into rounds

- 1 red onion, cut into chunks

- 8-10 cherry tomatoes

- 2 tablespoons olive oil

- 2 tablespoons balsamic vinegar

- 2 cloves garlic, minced

- 1 teaspoon dried Italian herbs (such as oregano, basil, thyme)

- Salt and pepper to taste

- Wooden skewers, soaked in water for 30 minutes

Instructions:

- In a bowl, combine olive oil, balsamic vinegar, minced garlic, dried Italian herbs, salt, and pepper to make the marinade.

- Thread chicken cubes and chopped vegetables onto the soaked wooden skewers, alternating between chicken and vegetables.

- Place the assembled skewers in a shallow dish and pour the marinade over them. Turn the skewers to coat evenly.

- Cover the dish and marinate in the refrigerator for at least 30 minutes, or up to 4 hours.

- Preheat the grill or grill pan over medium-high heat.

- Grill the skewers for 8-10 minutes, turning occasionally, until the chicken is cooked through and the vegetables are tender.

- Remove from the grill and let rest for a few minutes before serving.

- Serve the chicken and vegetable skewers hot alongside a side salad or whole grain for a complete meal.

- Enjoy these delicious and colorful skewers!

Health Benefits:

- These chicken and vegetable skewers are a great source of lean protein, vitamins, and minerals.

- Chicken provides high-quality protein and essential amino acids, while vegetables offer fiber, antioxidants, and bone-supportive nutrients.

- The dish is low in calories and saturated fat, making it suitable for a bone-healthy diet.

Preparation Time: Approximately 40 minutes (including marinating time).

5: Lentil and Vegetable Curry

Ingredients:

- 1 cup dried green lentils, rinsed and drained
- 4 cups vegetable broth
- 1 onion, chopped
- 2 carrots, diced
- 2 potatoes, diced
- 1 cup diced tomatoes (canned or fresh)
- 1 cup chopped spinach or kale
- 2 cloves garlic, minced
- 1 tablespoon grated ginger
- 2 tablespoons curry powder
- 1 teaspoon ground turmeric
- Salt and pepper to taste
- 1 tablespoon coconut oil
- Cooked brown rice for serving
- Optional garnish: chopped cilantro, lime wedges

Instructions:

- In a large pot, heat coconut oil over medium heat. Add chopped onion and cook until softened, about 5 minutes.
- Add minced garlic and grated ginger to the pot, and cook for another 1-2 minutes until fragrant.
- Stir in curry powder and ground turmeric, and cook for 1 minute to toast the spices.
- Add dried lentils, diced carrots, diced potatoes, diced tomatoes, and vegetable broth to the pot. Bring to a boil.
- Reduce heat to low, cover, and simmer for 20-25 minutes, or until lentils and vegetables are tender.
- Stir in chopped spinach or kale and cook for an additional 5 minutes until wilted.
- Season with salt and pepper to taste.
- Serve the lentil and vegetable curry over cooked brown rice.
- Garnish with chopped cilantro and serve with lime wedges, if desired.
- Enjoy this flavorful and nourishing curry!

Health Benefits:

- This lentil and vegetable curry is packed with plant-based protein, fiber, vitamins, and minerals.
- Lentils are rich in protein, iron, and folate, while vegetables provide essential nutrients like vitamin C, vitamin K, and antioxidants.
- Turmeric offers anti-inflammatory properties beneficial for bone health.

Preparation Time: Approximately 45 minutes.

6: Grilled Vegetable Quinoa Salad

Ingredients:

- 1 cup cooked quinoa
- 1 zucchini, sliced lengthwise
- 1 yellow squash, sliced lengthwise
- 1 red bell pepper, halved and seeded
- 1 red onion, sliced into rounds
- 1 cup cherry tomatoes
- 2 tablespoons olive oil
- 1 tablespoon balsamic vinegar

- 1 teaspoon dried Italian herbs (such as oregano, basil, thyme)
- Salt and pepper to taste
- 1/4 cup crumbled feta cheese
- 2 tablespoons chopped fresh basil
- Optional: balsamic glaze for drizzling

Instructions:

- Preheat the grill or grill pan over medium-high heat.
- In a bowl, whisk together olive oil, balsamic vinegar, dried Italian herbs, salt, and pepper to make the marinade.
- Brush the sliced zucchini, yellow squash, red bell pepper, and red onion with the marinade.
- Grill the vegetables for 3-4 minutes per side, or until tender and lightly charred.
- Remove the grilled vegetables from the grill and let cool slightly.
- Chop the grilled vegetables into bite-sized pieces and transfer to a large bowl.

- Add cooked quinoa, cherry tomatoes, crumbled feta cheese, and chopped fresh basil to the bowl with the grilled vegetables.
- Toss gently to combine all ingredients.
- Drizzle with balsamic glaze, if desired, before serving.
- Enjoy this vibrant and nutritious grilled vegetable quinoa salad!

Health Benefits:

- This grilled vegetable quinoa salad is rich in fiber, vitamins, and minerals.
- Quinoa provides protein and complex carbohydrates, while grilled vegetables offer antioxidants and bone-supportive nutrients.
- Olive oil and feta cheese provide healthy fats and calcium, respectively.

Preparation Time: Approximately 30 minutes.

7: Stuffed Portobello Mushrooms

Ingredients:

- 4 large portobello mushrooms, stems removed

- 1 cup cooked quinoa
- 1 cup cooked lentils
- 1 cup baby spinach, chopped
- 1/2 cup diced tomatoes
- 1/4 cup diced red onion
- 2 cloves garlic, minced
- 1 teaspoon dried Italian herbs (such as oregano, basil, thyme)
- Salt and pepper to taste
- 1/4 cup grated Parmesan cheese (optional)
- 2 tablespoons olive oil

Instructions:

- Preheat the oven to 375°F (190°C). Line a baking sheet with parchment paper.
- Place portobello mushrooms on the prepared baking sheet, gill side up.
- In a large bowl, combine cooked quinoa, cooked lentils, chopped baby spinach, diced tomatoes, diced red onion, minced garlic, dried Italian herbs, salt, and pepper.

- Spoon the quinoa and lentil mixture evenly into each portobello mushroom cap.

- Drizzle olive oil over the stuffed mushrooms.

- Bake in the preheated oven for 20-25 minutes, or until the mushrooms are tender and the filling is heated through.

- If using, sprinkle grated Parmesan cheese over the stuffed mushrooms during the last 5 minutes of baking.

- Remove from the oven and let cool for a few minutes before serving.

- Enjoy these flavorful and nutritious stuffed portobello mushrooms!

Health Benefits:

- These stuffed portobello mushrooms are rich in plant-based protein, fiber, vitamins, and minerals.

- Quinoa and lentils provide protein and essential nutrients for bone health, while spinach offers calcium and vitamin K.

- Portobello mushrooms are low in calories and provide additional vitamins and antioxidants.

Preparation Time: Approximately 35 minutes.

8: Lemon Herb Baked Chicken

Ingredients:

- 4 boneless, skinless chicken breasts
- 2 tablespoons olive oil
- 2 tablespoons lemon juice
- 2 cloves garlic, minced
- 1 teaspoon dried thyme
- 1 teaspoon dried rosemary
- 1 teaspoon dried oregano
- Salt and pepper to taste
- Lemon slices for garnish
- Fresh parsley for garnish

Instructions:

- Preheat the oven to 400°F (200°C). Line a baking dish with parchment paper.
- In a small bowl, whisk together olive oil, lemon juice, minced garlic, dried thyme, dried rosemary, dried oregano, salt, and pepper to make the marinade.
- Place chicken breasts in the prepared baking dish.

- Pour the marinade over the chicken breasts, turning to coat evenly.

- Arrange lemon slices on top of each chicken breast.

- Bake in the preheated oven for 20-25 minutes, or until the chicken is cooked through and juices run clear.

- Remove from the oven and let rest for a few minutes before serving.

- Garnish with fresh parsley before serving.

- Enjoy this juicy and flavorful lemon herb baked chicken!

Health Benefits:

- This lemon herb baked chicken is a great source of lean protein, vitamins, and minerals.

- Chicken breasts provide high-quality protein and essential amino acids necessary for bone health.

- Herbs like thyme, rosemary, and oregano offer antioxidants and anti-inflammatory properties.

Preparation Time: Approximately 30 minutes.

9: Broccoli and Mushroom Stir-Fry with Tofu

Ingredients:

- 1 block (14 oz) extra-firm tofu, pressed and cubed
- 2 tablespoons soy sauce (or tamari for gluten-free option)
- 2 tablespoons hoisin sauce
- 1 tablespoon sesame oil
- 2 cloves garlic, minced
- 1 teaspoon grated ginger
- 2 cups broccoli florets
- 2 cups sliced mushrooms (such as cremini or shiitake)
- 1 red bell pepper, sliced
- Cooked brown rice or quinoa for serving
- Optional garnish: sliced green onions, sesame seeds

Instructions:

- In a bowl, combine cubed tofu with soy sauce and let marinate for 15-20 minutes.
- In a small bowl, mix hoisin sauce and sesame oil to make the sauce.

- Heat a large skillet or wok over medium-high heat. Add marinated tofu and cook until golden brown on all sides, about 5-7 minutes. Remove tofu from the skillet and set aside.
- In the same skillet, add minced garlic and grated ginger. Stir-fry for 1 minute until fragrant.
- Add broccoli florets, sliced mushrooms, and sliced red bell pepper to the skillet. Stir-fry until vegetables are tender-crisp, about 5-7 minutes.
- Return cooked tofu to the skillet and pour the sauce over the tofu and vegetables. Toss to combine and heat through.
- Serve the broccoli and mushroom stir-fry over cooked brown rice or quinoa.
- Garnish with sliced green onions and sesame seeds, if desired.
- Enjoy this delicious and nutrient-packed stir-fry!

Health Benefits:

- This broccoli and mushroom stir-fry with tofu is loaded with plant-based protein, fiber, vitamins, and minerals.

- Tofu provides calcium and protein, while broccoli and mushrooms offer antioxidants, vitamins, and minerals essential for bone health.

- Brown rice or quinoa adds complex carbohydrates and additional fiber.

Preparation Time: Approximately 30 minutes.

10: Baked Sweet Potato with Chickpea and Spinach Salad

Ingredients:

- 2 large sweet potatoes
- 1 can (15 oz) chickpeas, rinsed and drained
- 2 cups fresh spinach leaves
- 1/4 cup diced red onion
- 1/4 cup chopped fresh parsley
- 2 tablespoons lemon juice
- 2 tablespoons olive oil
- 1 teaspoon ground cumin
- Salt and pepper to taste

Instructions:

- Preheat the oven to 400°F (200°C). Line a baking sheet with parchment paper.
- Scrub sweet potatoes and pierce each several times with a fork. Place on the prepared baking sheet and bake for 45-60 minutes, or until tender.
- In a large bowl, combine chickpeas, fresh spinach leaves, diced red onion, and chopped fresh parsley.
- In a small bowl, whisk together lemon juice, olive oil, ground cumin, salt, and pepper to make the dressing.
- Pour the dressing over the chickpea and spinach salad. Toss gently to coat.
- Once the sweet potatoes are cooked and slightly cooled, slice each one lengthwise without cutting all the way through.
- Fluff the insides of the sweet potatoes with a fork and top with chickpea and spinach salad.
- Serve immediately and enjoy this hearty and nutritious baked sweet potato!

Health Benefits:

- This baked sweet potato with chickpea and spinach salad is rich in fiber, protein, vitamins, and minerals.
- Sweet potatoes provide beta-carotene, while chickpeas offer plant-based protein and fiber. Spinach is a great source of calcium and vitamin K, important for bone health.

Preparation Time: Approximately 1 hour.

Osteoporosis Diet Snacks Recipes

1: Greek Yogurt Parfait

Ingredients:

- 1 cup plain Greek yogurt
- 1/2 cup mixed berries (such as strawberries, blueberries, raspberries)
- 1/4 cup granola
- 1 tablespoon honey or maple syrup (optional)
- Optional toppings: sliced almonds, chia seeds, flaxseeds

Instructions:

- In a serving glass or bowl, layer plain Greek yogurt, mixed berries, and granola.
- Drizzle honey or maple syrup over the top, if desired.
- Repeat the layers until the glass or bowl is filled.
- Sprinkle optional toppings such as sliced almonds, chia seeds, or flaxseeds on top.
- Serve immediately and enjoy this delicious and nutritious Greek yogurt parfait!

Health Benefits:

- This Greek yogurt parfait is rich in calcium, protein, probiotics, and antioxidants.
- Greek yogurt provides calcium and protein essential for bone health, while mixed berries offer vitamins, minerals, and antioxidants.
- Granola adds fiber and healthy fats, while optional toppings provide additional nutrients.

Preparation Time: Approximately 5 minutes.

2: Avocado Toast with Tomato

Ingredients:

- 2 slices whole grain bread
- 1 ripe avocado
- 1 medium tomato, sliced
- 1 tablespoon lemon juice
- Salt and pepper to taste
- Optional toppings: red pepper flakes, sesame seeds, microgreens

Instructions:

- Toast the slices of whole grain bread until golden brown.
- In a small bowl, mash the ripe avocado with lemon juice, salt, and pepper until smooth.
- Spread mashed avocado evenly on each slice of toasted bread.
- Top avocado toast with sliced tomatoes.
- Sprinkle optional toppings such as red pepper flakes, sesame seeds, or microgreens over the top.
- Serve immediately and enjoy this simple and nutritious avocado toast with tomato!

Health Benefits:

- This avocado toast with tomato is packed with fiber, healthy fats, vitamins, and minerals.
- Avocado provides monounsaturated fats and potassium, while whole grain bread offers complex carbohydrates and fiber.
- Tomatoes are rich in vitamin C, vitamin K, and antioxidants beneficial for bone health.

Preparation Time: Approximately 10 minutes.

3: Almond Butter and Banana Rice Cakes

Ingredients:

- 2 rice cakes (whole grain or brown rice)
- 2 tablespoons almond butter (or any nut or seed butter)
- 1 ripe banana, sliced
- Optional toppings: cinnamon, honey, chia seeds

Instructions:

- Spread almond butter evenly on each rice cake.
- Arrange sliced banana on top of the almond butter layer.

- Sprinkle optional toppings such as cinnamon, honey, or chia seeds over the banana slices.
- Serve immediately and enjoy these satisfying almond butter and banana rice cakes!

Health Benefits:

- These almond butter and banana rice cakes are rich in fiber, healthy fats, vitamins, and minerals.
- Almond butter provides calcium, magnesium, and vitamin E, while bananas offer potassium and vitamin B6.
- Whole grain rice cakes add complex carbohydrates and fiber, making this snack a nutritious choice for bone health.

Preparation Time: Approximately 5 minutes.

4: Veggie Sticks with Hummus

Ingredients:

- Assorted vegetable sticks (such as carrots, cucumber, bell peppers, celery)
- 1/4 cup hummus (store-bought or homemade)

Instructions:

- Wash and peel the vegetables as needed. Cut them into sticks or slices.
- Arrange the vegetable sticks on a plate or in a container.
- Serve with hummus for dipping.
- Enjoy these crunchy and nutritious veggie sticks with hummus as a satisfying snack!

Health Benefits:

- This snack is loaded with vitamins, minerals, fiber, and antioxidants.
- Vegetables provide essential nutrients like vitamin C, vitamin K, and potassium, which are beneficial for bone health.
- Hummus offers plant-based protein and healthy fats, making it a nutritious dip option.

Preparation Time: Approximately 10 minutes (depending on vegetable preparation).

5: Kale Chips

Ingredients:

- 1 bunch kale
- 1 tablespoon olive oil
- Salt and pepper to taste
- Optional: nutritional yeast, garlic powder, chili powder

Instructions:

- Preheat the oven to 300°F (150°C). Line a baking sheet with parchment paper.
- Wash the kale leaves and pat them dry with a paper towel.
- Remove the stems and tear the kale leaves into bite-sized pieces.
- In a large bowl, toss the kale pieces with olive oil, ensuring they are evenly coated.
- Arrange the kale pieces in a single layer on the prepared baking sheet.
- Season with salt, pepper, and any optional seasonings such as nutritional yeast, garlic powder, or chili powder.

- Bake in the preheated oven for 10-15 minutes, or until the kale chips are crisp but not burnt.
- Remove from the oven and let cool before serving.
- Enjoy these crispy and flavorful kale chips as a nutritious snack!

Health Benefits:

- Kale is rich in calcium, vitamin K, and other nutrients essential for bone health.
- Kale chips are a crunchy and delicious way to incorporate this nutrient-packed vegetable into your diet.
- Olive oil provides healthy fats, while seasonings add flavor without excess calories.

Preparation Time: Approximately 20 minutes.

6: Cottage Cheese with Pineapple

Ingredients:

- 1/2 cup low-fat cottage cheese
- 1/2 cup fresh pineapple chunks
- Optional: shredded coconut, chopped nuts

Instructions:

- In a small bowl, scoop the cottage cheese.
- Add fresh pineapple chunks on top of the cottage cheese.
- Sprinkle shredded coconut and chopped nuts over the cottage cheese and pineapple, if desired.
- Serve immediately and enjoy this creamy and refreshing cottage cheese with pineapple!

Health Benefits:

- Cottage cheese is an excellent source of protein and calcium, both of which are important for bone health.
- Fresh pineapple provides vitamin C and manganese, which support collagen production and bone formation.
- This snack is low in calories and provides a good balance of protein, carbohydrates, and healthy fats.

Preparation Time: Approximately 5 minutes.

7: Chia Seed Pudding

Ingredients:

- 1/4 cup chia seeds

- 1 cup unsweetened almond milk (or any milk of choice)
- 1 tablespoon maple syrup or honey (optional)
- 1/2 teaspoon vanilla extract
- Fresh fruit for topping (such as berries, sliced bananas)
- Optional toppings: chopped nuts, shredded coconut, cinnamon

Instructions:

- In a bowl or jar, combine chia seeds, unsweetened almond milk, maple syrup or honey (if using), and vanilla extract.
- Stir well to combine all ingredients.
- Cover and refrigerate the mixture for at least 2 hours or overnight, allowing the chia seeds to absorb the liquid and thicken.
- Stir the chia seed pudding before serving to ensure it has a creamy consistency.
- Serve the chia seed pudding topped with fresh fruit and any optional toppings of your choice.

- Enjoy this nutritious and satisfying chia seed pudding as a snack!

Health Benefits:

- Chia seeds are rich in calcium, magnesium, and phosphorus, which are essential for bone health.
- They also provide omega-3 fatty acids and fiber.
- Unsweetened almond milk adds calcium and vitamin D without added sugars.
- This snack is low in calories and high in nutrients, making it a great choice for bone health.

Preparation Time: Approximately 5 minutes (plus chilling time).

8: Edamame Hummus with Whole Grain Crackers

Ingredients:

- 1 cup shelled edamame (thawed if frozen)
- 1/4 cup tahini
- 2 tablespoons lemon juice
- 1 clove garlic, minced
- 2 tablespoons olive oil

- Salt and pepper to taste

- Whole grain crackers for serving

Instructions:

- In a food processor, combine shelled edamame, tahini, lemon juice, minced garlic, olive oil, salt, and pepper.

- Blend until smooth, scraping down the sides of the food processor as needed, until the desired consistency is reached.

- If the hummus is too thick, you can add a little water or more olive oil to thin it out.

- Transfer the edamame hummus to a serving bowl.

- Serve with whole grain crackers for dipping.

- Enjoy this flavorful and nutritious edamame hummus as a satisfying snack!

Health Benefits:

- Edamame is a good source of plant-based protein, calcium, and vitamin K, all of which are important for bone health.

- Tahini adds healthy fats and additional protein, while lemon juice provides vitamin C.
- Whole grain crackers offer fiber and complex carbohydrates, making this snack balanced and nutritious.

Preparation Time: Approximately 10 minutes.

9: Spinach and Feta Stuffed Mushrooms

Ingredients:

- 8 large button mushrooms
- 1 cup fresh spinach, chopped
- 1/4 cup crumbled feta cheese
- 1 clove garlic, minced
- 1 tablespoon olive oil
- Salt and pepper to taste

Instructions:

- Preheat the oven to 375°F (190°C). Line a baking sheet with parchment paper.
- Remove the stems from the mushrooms and gently scoop out some of the gills to create a hollow space.

- In a skillet, heat olive oil over medium heat. Add minced garlic and chopped spinach, and sauté until the spinach wilts, about 2-3 minutes.
- Remove the skillet from heat and stir in crumbled feta cheese. Season with salt and pepper to taste.
- Spoon the spinach and feta mixture into each mushroom cap, pressing down gently to fill.
- Place the stuffed mushrooms on the prepared baking sheet.
- Bake in the preheated oven for 15-20 minutes, or until the mushrooms are tender and the filling is heated through.
- Remove from the oven and let cool for a few minutes before serving.
- Enjoy these delicious spinach and feta stuffed mushrooms as a nutritious snack!

Health Benefits:

- Spinach is a rich source of calcium, vitamin K, and magnesium, all of which are important for bone health.
- Feta cheese adds calcium and protein to the snack.

- Mushrooms provide vitamin D when exposed to sunlight, and they are low in calories and high in antioxidants.

Preparation Time: Approximately 25 minutes.

10: Almond and Date Energy Balls

Ingredients:

- 1 cup pitted dates
- 1 cup raw almonds
- 2 tablespoons unsweetened cocoa powder
- 1 tablespoon chia seeds
- 1/2 teaspoon vanilla extract
- Pinch of salt
- Optional: shredded coconut for coating

Instructions:

- In a food processor, combine pitted dates, raw almonds, cocoa powder, chia seeds, vanilla extract, and a pinch of salt.
- Process the mixture until it forms a sticky dough-like consistency.

- Scoop out tablespoon-sized portions of the mixture and roll them into balls using your hands.

- If desired, roll the energy balls in shredded coconut to coat.

- Place the energy balls on a baking sheet lined with parchment paper.

- Refrigerate the energy balls for at least 30 minutes to firm up.

- Once chilled, transfer the energy balls to an airtight container for storage.

- Enjoy these almond and date energy balls as a convenient and nutritious snack!

Health Benefits:

- Dates are a natural sweetener and provide fiber, potassium, and magnesium.

- Almonds are rich in calcium, protein, and healthy fats. Chia seeds add omega-3 fatty acids and additional fiber.

- These energy balls are nutrient-dense and provide a quick energy boost.

Preparation Time: Approximately 15 minutes.

CONCLUSION

The Osteoporosis Diet Cookbook offers a comprehensive and delicious approach to supporting bone health through nutrition. By incorporating nutrient-rich foods into our daily meals and snacks, we can nourish our bodies with the essential vitamins, minerals, and antioxidants needed for strong and resilient bones.

From hearty breakfasts to satisfying dinners and everything in between, this cookbook provides a wide array of flavorful recipes designed specifically to promote bone health.

Whether it's enjoying a refreshing green smoothie packed with calcium-rich greens or savoring a comforting bowl of lentil soup brimming with protein and fiber, each recipe is crafted with care to support your osteoporosis diet journey.

With clear instructions, helpful tips, and nutritional information provided for each recipe, this cookbook empowers readers to make informed choices about their dietary habits and take proactive steps toward maintaining optimal bone health.

By embracing the principles of the osteoporosis diet and incorporating these delicious recipes into your meal planning, you can embark on a journey toward stronger bones and overall well-being.

Let the Osteoporosis Diet Cookbook be your guide to a flavorful and nourishing culinary experience that supports your bone health for years to come.

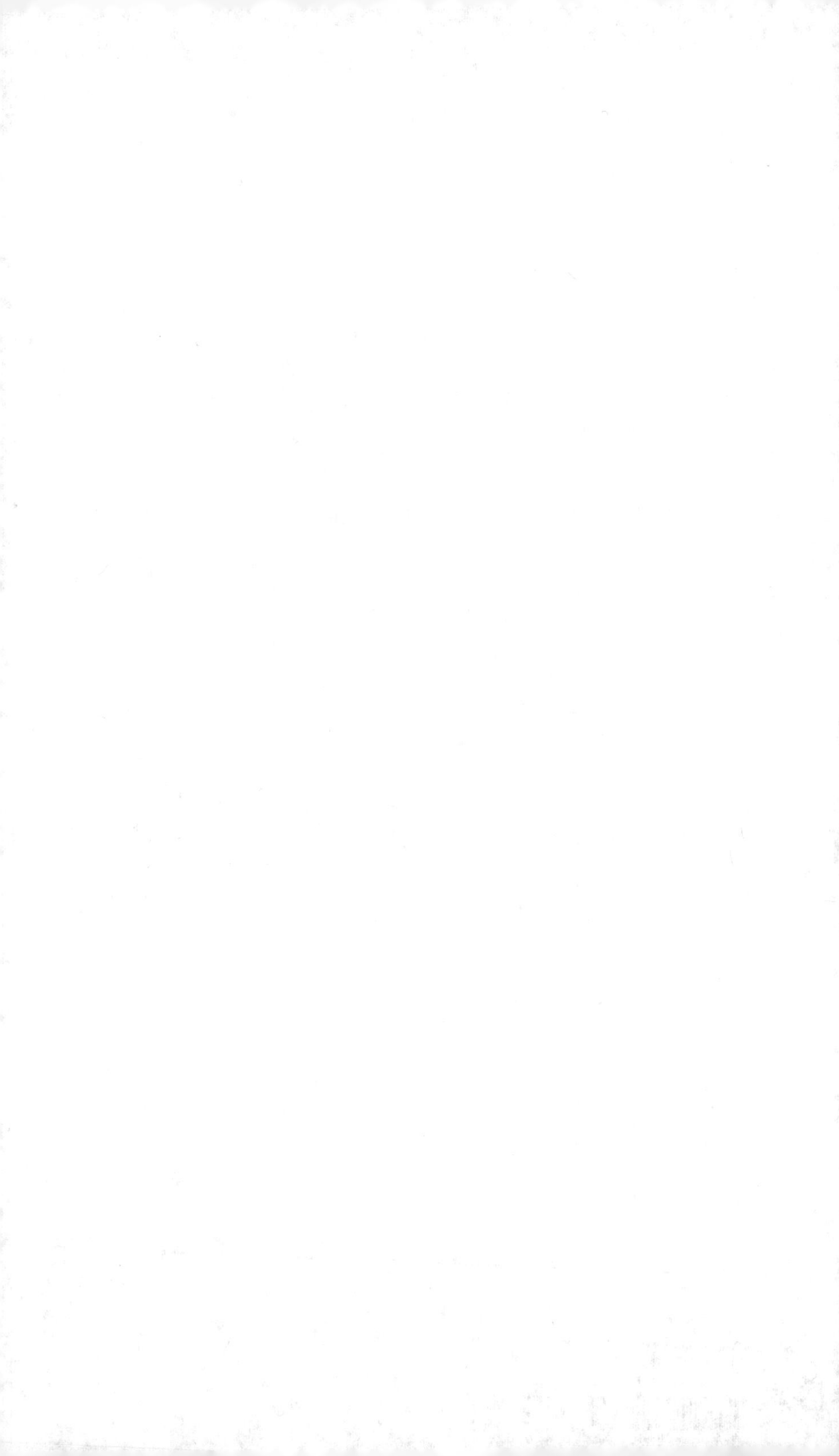